# MEDITERRANEAN WELLNESS RECIPES FOR COUPLES

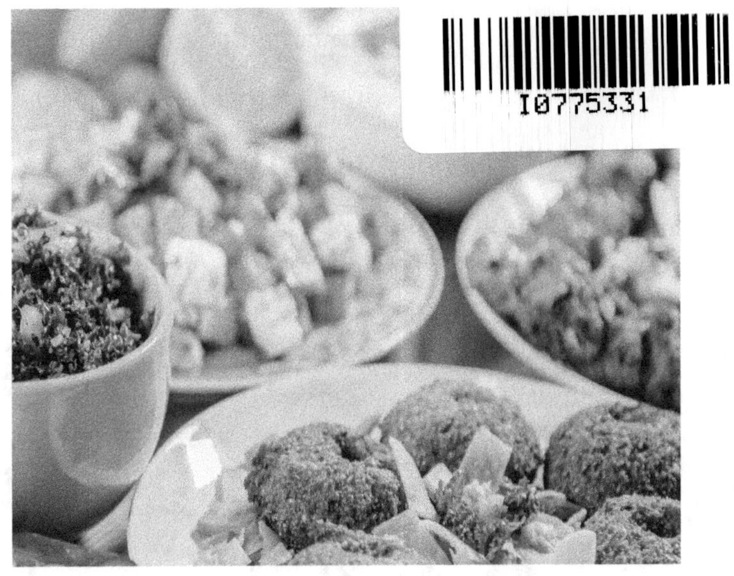

*A comprehensive guide on cooking delights for two.*

Lela B. Gillete

1

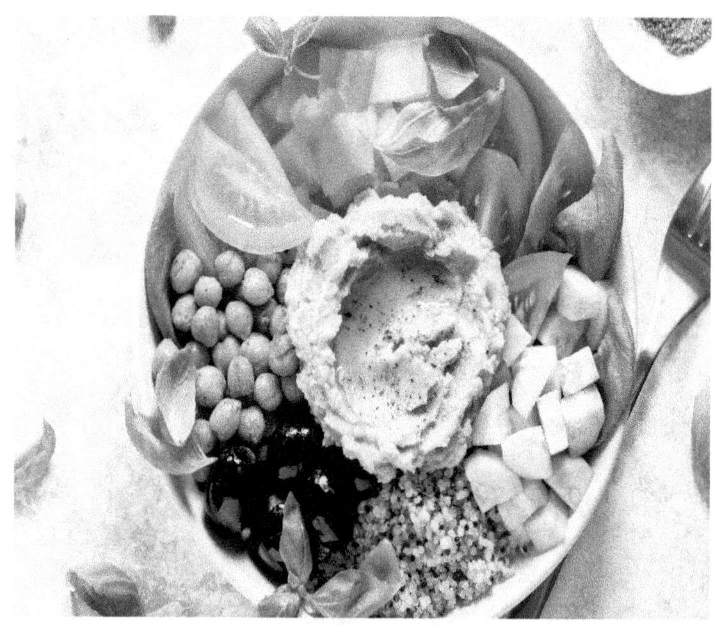

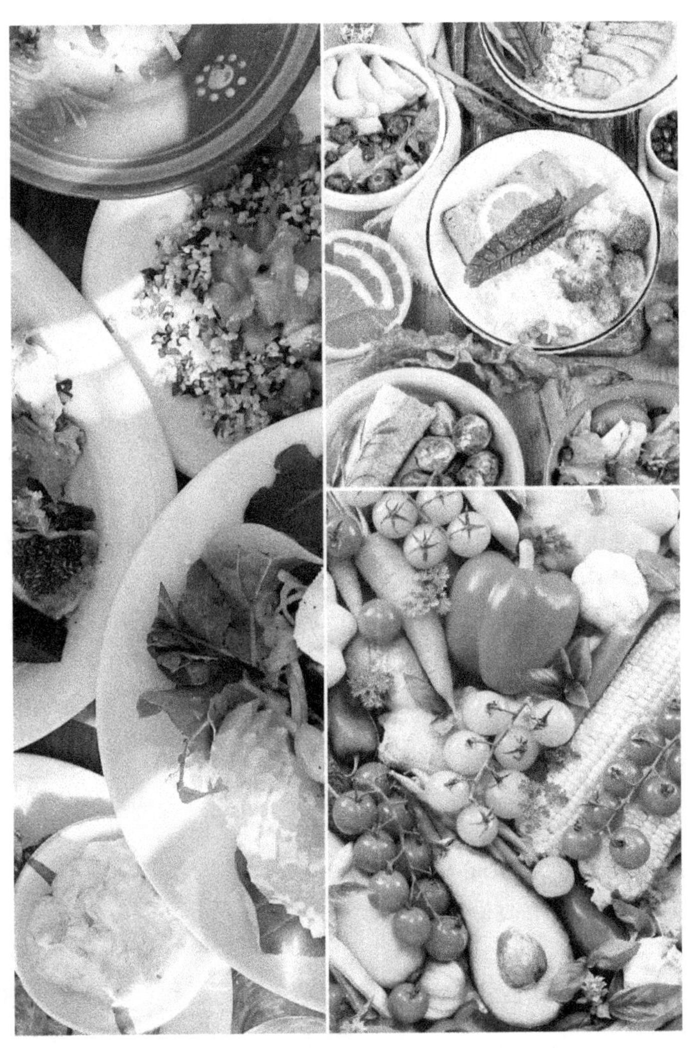

# Table of Contents

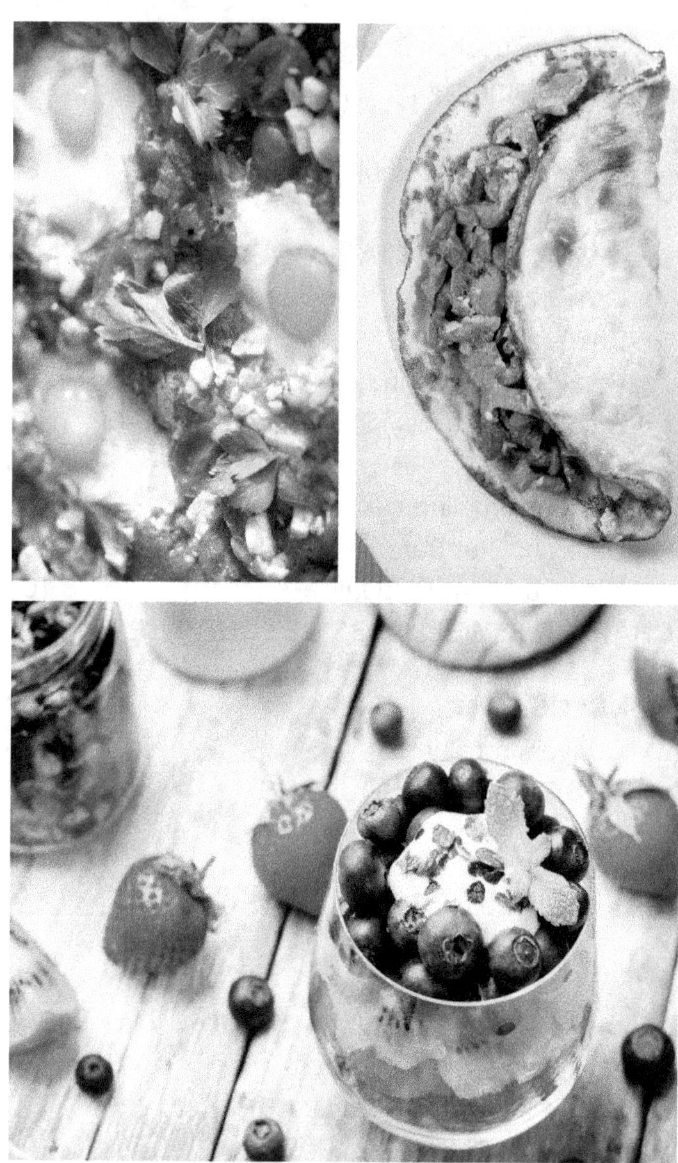

## INTRODUCTION

Rachel and David lived in the lovely neighborhood of Oak Grove, tucked among calm streets and swaying trees, a couple linked by their love for each other and a shared enthusiasm for relishing life's simple pleasures. Their experience with Mediterranean Wellness Recipes for Couples did not begin with a resounding revelation; rather, it gradually crept into their life in subtle, transforming ways.

Rachel, an ambitious graphic designer with a voracious appetite for new experiences, came upon the book while perusing a local bookshop. Its cover enticed her with vivid pictures of fresh fruit and sun-soaked landscapes. She knew it was something she and David could explore together, intrigued by the promise of wellbeing and the attraction of Mediterranean cuisine.

As she turned the pages, each dish seemed to open a door to a world of flavor and heritage. The simplicity of the components, along with the promise of delectable tastes, piqued her interest. She saw herself and David not just sharing meals, but also beginning on a shared adventure of discovery packed with fragrant spices, nutritious foods, and the promise of a better, more connected existence.

Rachel carried the book home with a twinkle in her eye, and that evening, while they lounged in their warm kitchen, she presented her acquired treasure. The book's approachability intrigued David, a software engineer with a penchant for accuracy and detail. The recipes' simplicity appealed to his pragmatic character, and the promise of health spoke to his quest for a balanced living.

They began their Mediterranean trip together, beginning with a simple breakfast of Greek yogurt and honey, a meal that seemed almost too basic yet had an air of pleasure. Rachel and David sensed a subtle change as they relished the creamy yogurt drizzled with golden honey and sprinkled with broken almonds. It was an unconscious connection established by the act of sharing a moment of pure gastronomic pleasure.

Weeks passed, and their kitchen became a canvas on which they painted tastes inspired by the Mediterranean palette. They savored the crispness of Greek salads, swooned over the perfume of lemon herb chicken, and marveled at the exquisite sweetness of homemade baklava. Each dish was a chapter in their narrative, a monument to their blossoming friendship and shared dedication to wellbeing.

But it wasn't just the food; it was the discussions that developed over chopping boards, the laughter that resonated as they experimented with new tastes, and the warmth that wrapped them as they enjoyed each other's company that made it so special. The book became more than simply a compilation of recipes; it became a catalyst for deeper relationships, a visible manifestation of their dedication to nurturing not just their bodies but also their relationship.

Rachel and David learned, via their culinary adventure, that the core of Mediterranean health was more than simply food; it was a way of life, a symphony of conscious eating, shared experiences, and a celebration of togetherness. They discovered that they enjoyed not just healthier, more tasty meals, but also a lifestyle that stressed connection, balance, and pleasure.

Their journey with Mediterranean Wellness Recipes for Couples was about adopting a concept that encouraged them to embrace life's moments, treasure their time together, and relish the simple joys found in a shared meal, rather than mastering difficult recipes or sticking to rigorous diets.

Rachel and David realized their voyage had only just started as they glanced over the well-worn pages of the book, stained with spices and memories. Their narrative, delicately intertwined with Mediterranean tastes and experiences, was a monument to the transformational power of food and love, reflected through the fragrances of their kitchen and the warmth of their shared smiles.

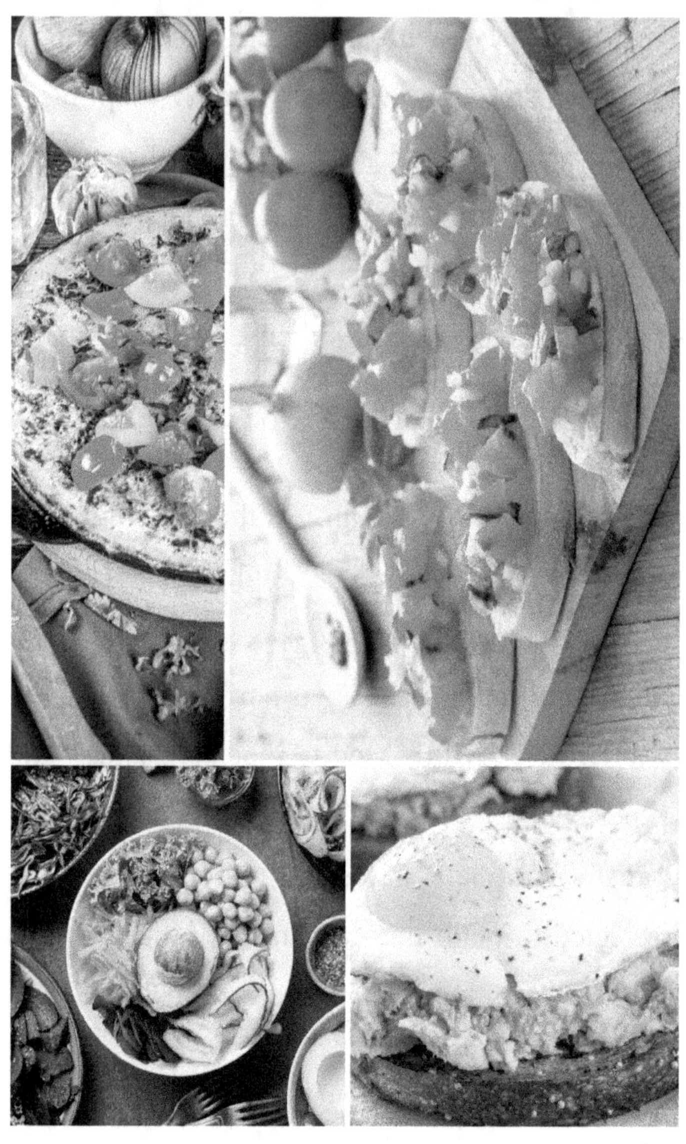

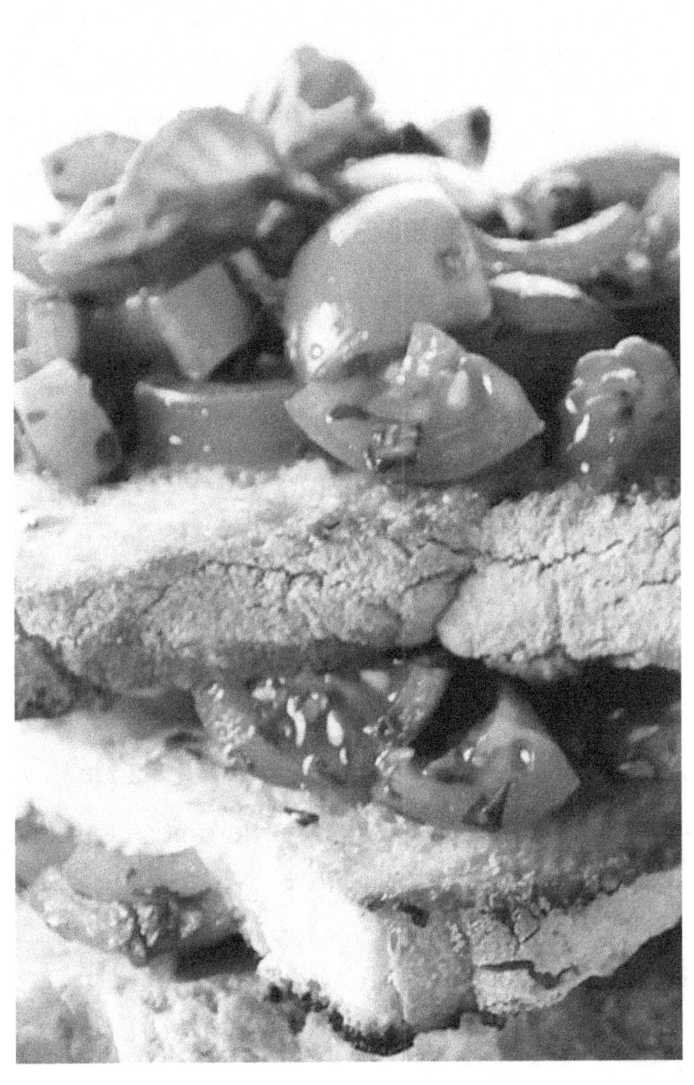

# CHAPTER 1: UNDERSTANDING MEDITERRANEAN WELLNESS.

The Mediterranean way of life stands out like a bright mosaic in the broad fabric of wellbeing, a combination of tastes, customs, and behaviors that have lasted the test of time. But what is Mediterranean wellness, and why has it captured the hearts and taste buds of people all over the world? Let's go on an adventure to discover the essence of this comprehensive approach to well-being.

At its foundation, Mediterranean health is a way of life that includes not just what we eat but also how we live, connect, and achieve balance. It is based on the habits of Mediterranean nations such as Greece, Italy, and Spain, where people have long embraced a way of life that balances health, happiness, and social living.

The Mediterranean diet, a gourmet treasure trove famous for its abundance of fresh, whole foods, is one of the cornerstones of this health strategy. It's a diet rich in vibrant fruits and vegetables, heart-healthy olive oil, whole grains, lean meats like fish and chicken, and a dash of nuts and seeds. Its meals are produced from nature's abundance and are brimming with nutrients and tastes.

But it's not just about the ingredients; it's about how they combine, a celebration of balance and moderation. The Mediterranean diet is not restrictive; it is inclusive, allowing for genuine enjoyment of life's joys. It's about enjoying the tastes of a ripe tomato, basking in the richness of olive oil, and cherishing the conviviality of shared meals.

The key to this diet's popularity is its remarkable health advantages. A Mediterranean diet has been proven in studies to decrease the risk of heart disease, reduce inflammation, boost brain health, and lead to a longer, more vibrant life. It's more than just a diet; it's a plan for cultivating both physical and mental well-being.

But, beyond the plate, Mediterranean health embraces many facets of life. It's about living an active lifestyle, a joyful dance of movement and relaxation. Daily physical exercise, whether it's a leisurely walk along the beach or a game of bocce in the park, is woven into the fabric of Mediterranean life.

The focus on social relationships and community is also significant. Meals are a celebration and an occasion for family and friends to congregate, exchange tales, and form strong ties in Mediterranean culture. This social attitude generates a feeling of belonging and emotional well-being, which is an essential component of the Mediterranean way of life.

Furthermore, Mediterranean health emphasizes mindfulness, or the discipline of being present in the moment. Whether it's sharing a meal with loved ones, meditating by the sea, or just taking in a sunset, mindfulness pervades all aspects of life, cultivating appreciation and mental clarity.

In essence, Mediterranean wellness is a concept, a mild guiding principle that promotes a healthy combination of nutrition, activity, social connection, and mindfulness. It's about enjoying life's pleasures while respecting the body, making relationships, and finding balance in an ever-changing environment.

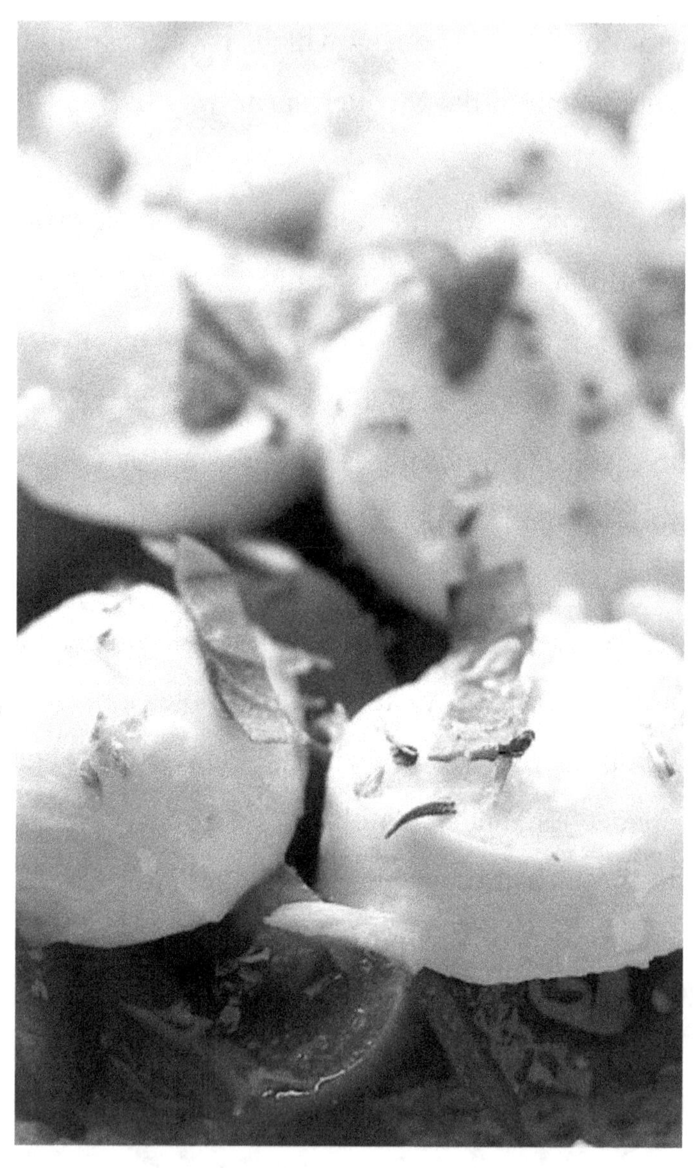

# CHAPTER 2: BREAKFAST DELIGHTS.

## Omelete

**Ingredients:**

- 3 large eggs.
- 1 tablespoon butter or olive oil.
- 1/4 cup shredded cheese (cheddar, Swiss, or your choice).
- 1 tablespoon chopped fresh herbs (parsley, chives, or basil).
- Salt and pepper to taste.

**Instructions:**

1. Prepare the ingredients: Break the eggs into a mixing dish and whisk until fully blended. Season with salt and pepper to taste.
2. Preheat and prepare: Melt butter in a nonstick pan over medium heat. Pour in

the butter or olive oil, making sure it covers the bottom of the pan evenly and melts.

3. Pour and Cook: Once the butter or oil is heated, pour in the whisked eggs. As the edges begin to solidify, use a spatula to gently press them towards the center, enabling the raw eggs to flow to the edges.

4. Add Fillings: When the omelet is mostly done but still little runny on top, sprinkle shredded cheese evenly over one side of it. On top of the cheese, sprinkle it with chopped herbs.

5. Fold and Finish: Carefully fold the omelet in half to cover the cheese and herbs using a spatula. Cook for 30 seconds to a minute more, or until the cheese is fully melted and the omelet is cooked through but still moist.

6. Serve: Slide the omelet onto a platter and top with more herbs or a sprinkling of cheese, if preferred. Serve immediately and enjoy!

## Greek yogurt parfait.

**Ingredients:**

- 1 cup Greek yogurt.
- 1/2 cup granola (homemade or store-bought).
- 1 cup mixed berries (strawberries, blueberries, raspberries).
- 2 tablespoons honey or maple syrup.
- 1/4 cup chopped nuts (almonds, walnuts, or pecans).
- Fresh mint leaves for garnish (optional).

**Instructions:**

1. Prepare the Berries: Wash the berries well and, if used, slice the strawberries.

Toss them lightly in a dish with honey or maple syrup for extra sweetness.

2. Layering: Use a glass or a parfait dish for this. Begin by spooning Greek yogurt into the bottom of the glass.

3. Add Granola: Sprinkle granola on top of the yogurt. This gives the parfait crunch and texture.

4. Berries: Place a layer of honey-coated mixed berries on top of the granola.

5. Continue Layering: Layer yogurt, granola, and berries until you reach the top of the glass, concluding with a layer of berries on top.

6. Finishing Touches: For extra texture and richness, sprinkle chopped nuts over the last layer of berries.

7. Garnish and serve: For a flash of color and taste, garnish the parfait with a sprig of fresh mint leaves. Enjoy your

delicious Greek Yogurt Parfait right now!

## Shakshuka

**Ingredients:**

- 2 tablespoons of olive oil.
- 1 onion, finely chopped.
- 3 cloves garlic, minced.
- 1 red bell pepper, diced.
- 1 yellow bell pepper, diced.
- 1 teaspoon ground cumin.
- 1 teaspoon smoked paprika.
- 1/2 teaspoon ground cayenne pepper (adjust to taste).
- 1 teaspoon ground coriander (optional).
- 1 can (14 oz) diced tomatoes.
- 1 can (14 oz) tomato sauce or puree.
- Salt and pepper to taste.
- 4-6 large eggs.

- Fresh parsley or cilantro, chopped (for garnish).
- Crumbled feta cheese or goat cheese (optional, for serving).
- Crusty bread or pita (for serving).

**Instructions:**

1. Sauté Aromatics: In a large skillet or cast-iron pan, heat olive oil over medium heat. Sauté the chopped onions for 3-4 minutes, or until they begin to soften. Cook for 1 minute more, or until the garlic is fragrant.

2. Stir in the chopped red and yellow bell peppers and spices. Cook for 5 minutes, or until they soften somewhat. Combine the cumin, smoked paprika, cayenne pepper, and ground coriander (if using) in a mixing bowl. Mix the spices into the vegetables well.

3.  Tomato Base: Combine the chopped tomatoes and tomato sauce or puree in a mixing bowl. Season to taste with salt and pepper. Bring the mixture to a boil and cook for approximately 10-15 minutes, or until slightly thickened.

4.  Make Egg Wells: Make little wells or indentations in the tomato-pepper mixture with a spoon. In each indentation, crack an egg. Season the eggs with salt and pepper to taste.

5.  Poach the Eggs: Cover the pan with a lid and cook the eggs for 8-10 minutes, or until the egg whites are set but the yolks are still somewhat runny. The cooking time may vary based on how you like your eggs.

6.  Garnish and Serve: Remove the pan from the heat after the eggs are done to your preference. To add some freshness, sprinkle with chopped parsley or

cilantro. Serve the Shakshuka straight from the pan, spooning out the eggs with some of the delicious tomato-pepper sauce. Optionally, top with crumbled feta or goat cheese for extra richness. Dip with crusty bread or warm pita bread.

## Avocado toast.

**Ingredients:**

1. 2 slices of your favorite bread (sourdough, whole grain, or multigrain).
2. 1 ripe avocado.
3. 1 tablespoon lemon juice.
4. Salt and pepper to taste.
5. Red pepper flakes (optional).
6. Optional toppings: cherry tomatoes, sliced radishes, microgreens, poached or fried egg, crumbled feta cheese, or sliced cucumber.

**Instructions:**

1. Toast the Bread: Toast the bread pieces until they are crisp. Place aside.

2. Cut the ripe avocado in half, remove the pit, and scoop out the flesh into a dish. With a fork, mash the avocado until it reaches the desired consistency (smooth or slightly chunky).

3. Season the Avocado: Mix the lemon juice into the mashed avocado. The lemon juice provides flavor while also preventing the avocado from browning too rapidly. Season the avocado mash with salt and pepper to taste. For a dash of spice, add a sprinkle of red pepper flakes.

4. Assemble the Avocado Toast: Evenly distribute the mashed avocado over the toasted bread pieces.

5. Add Toppings: This is your chance to be creative! Add any of your preferred

toppings to the avocado toast. Cherry tomatoes, radishes, microgreens, a poached or fried egg, crumbled feta cheese, or sliced cucumber are all good choices. Toppings may be mixed and matched to suit your tastes.

6. Serve and Enjoy: Your avocado toast is ready to eat after you've added your favorite toppings. Serve it right away for a delicious and healthy breakfast, brunch, or snack.

## Breakfast bowl.

**Ingredients:**

1. 1 cup cooked quinoa or brown rice.
2. 2 eggs.
3. 1 ripe avocado, sliced.
4. 1/2 cup cherry tomatoes, halved.

5. 1/4 cup diced red bell pepper.

6. 1/4 cup diced cucumber.

7. 1/4 cup sliced radishes.

8. Handful of baby spinach or arugula.

9. 1 tablespoon of olive oil.

10. Salt and pepper to taste.

11. Optional toppings: sliced green onions, sesame seeds, crumbled feta cheese, hot sauce, or a drizzle of balsamic glaze.

## Instructions:

1. Begin by cooking the quinoa or brown rice according to package directions. When it's done, fluff it up and distribute it equally among serving dishes to form the basis of your breakfast bowl.

2. Sauté Vegetables: Heat olive oil in a pan over medium heat. Cook for a few minutes, until the red bell pepper is somewhat softened. Cook for another minute, or until the cherry tomatoes

begin to soften. Set aside after removing from the heat.

3. Cook the Eggs: In the same pan, cook or scramble the eggs to your liking. While cooking, season with salt and pepper to taste.

4. Assemble the Breakfast Bowl: Begin by placing the cooked quinoa or brown rice as the basis of your breakfast bowl. Sautéed bell peppers and tomatoes come first, followed by sliced avocado, diced cucumber, sliced radishes, and a handful of baby spinach or arugula.

5. Place the Cooked Eggs on Top: Place the cooked eggs on top of the bowl.

6. Finish with optional toppings such as sliced green onions, sesame seeds, crumbled feta cheese, a sprinkle of spicy sauce for a kick, or a spray of balsamic glaze for added flavor.

7. Serve and Enjoy: Your filling and healthy Breakfast Bowl is now ready to eat! For a great start to your day, combine the ingredients or enjoy each component individually.

## Style frittata.

**Ingredients:**

- 8 large eggs.
- 1/4 cup milk or cream.
- 1 tablespoon of olive oil.
- 1 small onion, diced.
- 1 bell pepper (any color), diced.
- 1 cup chopped spinach or kale.
- 1 cup sliced mushrooms.
- 1/2 cup grated cheese (cheddar, mozzarella, or your choice).
- Salt and pepper to taste.
- Fresh herbs (parsley, basil, or thyme) for garnish.

**Instructions:**

1. Preheat the oven to 350 degrees Fahrenheit (175 degrees Celsius).

2. Prepare the ingredients: Whisk together the eggs and milk or cream in a mixing dish until thoroughly blended. Season with salt and pepper to taste. Place aside.

3. Sauté Vegetables: In an oven-safe pan over medium heat, heat olive oil. Mix in the diced onions and bell peppers. 3-4 minutes, or until they start to soften. Cook for another 2-3 minutes, or until the sliced mushrooms begin to brown. Cook until the spinach or kale has wilted.

4. Pour in the egg mixture and equally distribute the sautéed veggies in the skillet. Pour the whisked eggs over the veggies, covering the whole surface.

enable it to simmer for 3-4 minutes on the burner to enable the edges to firm.

5. Add Cheese and Bake: Evenly distribute grated cheese over the top of the frittata. Place the pan in a preheated oven and bake for 12-15 minutes, or until the eggs are set in the center and the top is gently brown.

6. Garnish and Serve: When finished, take the pan from the oven (use oven mitts, it'll be hot!). Allow for a few minutes of cooling before serving. To enhance flavor and freshness, top with freshly chopped herbs.

7. To serve, cut the frittata into wedges straight off the griddle. It may be served hot, warm, or cold, making it a flexible meal at any time of day.

# Breakfast bruschetta

**Ingredients:**

- 4 slices of crusty bread (baguette or Italian bread).
- 4 large eggs.
- 1 avocado, sliced.
- 1 cup cherry tomatoes, halved.
- 1/4 cup chopped fresh basil.
- 2 tablespoons of olive oil.
- 1 garlic clove, peeled.
- Salt and pepper to taste.
- Optional toppings: crumbled feta cheese, chopped chives, or hot sauce.

**Instructions:**

1. Preheat the oven to 375 degrees F (190 degrees C). Toast the bread pieces on a

baking pan for approximately 5-7 minutes, or until they're gently brown and crispy. After removing from the oven, set aside.

2. Make the toppings: In a mixing dish, combine the cherry tomatoes, basil, and olive oil. Season to taste with salt and pepper. Set aside after gently tossing to combine.

3. Cook the eggs: Heat a tablespoon of olive oil in a nonstick pan over medium heat. Crack the eggs into the pan and cook until done to your liking (fried or scrambled). While the eggs are frying, season them with salt and pepper.

4. Garlic Bread massage: Gently massage the peeled garlic clove over the toasted bread pieces. This imparts a mild garlic taste to the bread.

5. Assemble the Bruschetta: Place avocado slices on top of the garlic-rubbed bread.

Spread the tomato and basil mixture on top of the avocado. Place a cooked egg on top of each bruschetta.

6. Optional Toppings: For added taste, serve with crumbled feta cheese, chopped chives, or a dash of spicy sauce.

7. Arrange the Breakfast Bruschetta on a tray or individual plates to serve. If preferred, garnish with more fresh basil leaves. Serve right away while the bread is still warm and the eggs are still heated.

# CHAPTER 3:LUNCHTIME INDULGENCES.

## Chicken salad

**Ingredients:**

- 2 cups cooked chicken, shredded or diced.
- 1/2 cup celery, finely chopped.

- 1/4 cup red onion, finely chopped.

- 1/2 cup grapes, halved.

- 1/4 cup toasted almonds or pecans, chopped (optional).

- 1/3 cup mayonnaise.

- 2 tablespoons of Greek yogurt or sour cream.

- 1 tablespoon lemon juice.

- 1 teaspoon Dijon mustard.

- Salt and pepper to taste.

- Lettuce leaves or bread/rolls for serving.

**Instructions:**

1. Poach chicken breasts in boiling water for around 15-20 minutes until cooked through if you don't have prepared chicken on hand. Allow to cool before slicing or chopping the cooked chicken.

2. Finely slice the celery and red onion, then cut the grapes in half. If using nuts, roast them for a few minutes in a dry pan

over medium heat until aromatic and lightly browned. Once cooled, chop them.

3. To make the dressing, whisk together mayonnaise, Greek yogurt or sour cream, lemon juice, Dijon mustard, salt, and pepper in a mixing bowl until thoroughly blended. Season to enjoy with pepper as well as salt.

4. To make the salad, combine the cooked chicken, celery, red onion, grapes, and toasted almonds (if using) in a large mixing dish. Pour the dressing over the ingredients and gently toss until equally covered.

5. Chill and serve: Refrigerate the chicken salad for at least 30 minutes to allow the flavors to mingle. This also enables it to cool, which improves the flavor.

6. Serve the chicken salad on lettuce leaves or as a sandwich filling on bread or buns.

It's also wonderful as a light dinner or snack on its own or with crackers.

## Falafel wraps with tzatziki

**Ingredients:**

**For Falafel:**

- 1 can (15 oz) chickpeas, drained and rinsed.
- 1/2 small onion, roughly chopped.
- 2 cloves garlic, minced.
- 1/4 cup fresh parsley, chopped.
- 1/4 cup fresh cilantro, chopped.
- 1 teaspoon ground cumin.
- 1 teaspoon ground coriander.
- 1/2 teaspoon baking powder.
- 3-4 tablespoons all-purpose flour or chickpea flour.
- Salt and pepper to taste.
- Oil for frying.

**For Tzatziki:**

- 1 cup Greek yogurt.
- 1/2 cucumber, grated and drained.
- 1-2 cloves garlic, minced.
- 1 tablespoon fresh dill, chopped.
- 1 tablespoon lemon juice.
- Salt and pepper to taste.

**For Wraps:**

- Pita bread or wraps.
- Lettuce leaves.
- Sliced tomatoes.
- Sliced red onions.
- Sliced cucumbers.
- Optional: Hummus or tahini sauce for spreading.

**Instructions:**

**Falafel:**

1. Make the falafel mixture by combining chickpeas, onion, garlic, parsley, cilantro, cumin, coriander, baking powder, flour, salt, and pepper in a food processor. Pulse the mixture until it is thoroughly blended but still somewhat gritty. If the mixture is too moist, add extra flour to bind it.

2. Scoop up pieces of the mixture and form into little balls or patties. Place them on a baking sheet lined with parchment paper.

3. Fry the falafel in a frying pan over medium heat. Fry the falafel balls in batches for 3-4 minutes each side, or until golden brown and crispy on the exterior. Remove and pat dry with paper towels.

**Tzatziki:**

1. To create Tzatziki, add Greek yogurt, grated cucumber (drain excess liquid), minced garlic, chopped dill, lemon juice, salt, and pepper in a mixing bowl. Combine thoroughly. Place in the refrigerator until ready to use.

2. Prepare the wrappings: Warm up the pita or wraps. Spread the bread with hummus or tahini sauce (if using).

3. Assemble Wraps: On the bread, layer lettuce leaves, sliced tomatoes, onions, and cucumbers. Fill each wrap with 2-3 falafel balls or patties.

4. Drizzle with Tzatziki: Drizzle the falafel with a large quantity of tzatziki sauce. Add extra fresh herbs or a splash of lemon juice if desired.

5. Fold and Serve: Fold the wrap's sides and roll it securely. If necessary, cover

with parchment paper or foil. Serve the falafel wraps right away and enjoy!

## Veggie pizza

**Ingredients:**

**For Pizza Dough:**

- 2 1/4 cups all-purpose flour.
- 1 packet (2 1/4 teaspoons) active dry yeast.
- 1 teaspoon sugar.
- 1 teaspoon salt.
- 1 cup warm water.
- 2 tablespoons of olive oil.

**For Pizza Toppings:**

- 1/2 cup pizza sauce or marinara sauce
- 1 cup shredded mozzarella cheese.

- Assorted vegetables (sliced bell peppers, sliced onions, sliced mushrooms, sliced tomatoes, spinach leaves, olives, etc.).
- 1/4 cup grated Parmesan cheese (optional).
- Fresh basil leaves for garnish (optional).

**Instructions:**

**Pizza Dough:**

1. Activate the yeast: Combine warm water, sugar, and yeast in a small basin. Allow it to settle for 5-10 minutes, or until the mixture gets frothy.

2. Combine the flour and salt in a large mixing dish. In a mixing dish, combine the yeast mixture and olive oil. Mix until a dough forms. Knead the dough on a lightly floured surface for 5-7 minutes, or until smooth and elastic.

3. First Rise: place the dough in a lightly oiled mixing basin, cover with a clean

kitchen towel or plastic wrap, and set aside in a warm location to rise for 1-1.5 hours, or until doubled in size.

4. Prepare the Oven: Preheat the oven to 450°F (230°C). Place your pizza stone in the oven to warm as well.

**Assembling and Baking:**

1. Make the Pizza: Punch down the rising dough and roll it out into your preferred pizza shape (round, rectangular, etc.) on a lightly floured surface. Place the rolled-out dough on a parchment-lined pizza pan or baking sheet.

2. Spread the pizza sauce evenly over the dough, leaving a little border for the crust. Shredded mozzarella cheese should be sprinkled on top of the sauce.

3. Veggies on top: Arrange your preferred veggies on top of the cheese. Feel free to pile them up thick.

4. Bake the pizza in a preheated oven. Bake for 12-15 minutes, or until the crust has become golden brown and the cheese has melted.

5. Finish and Serve: When the pizza is done, take it from the oven. For added taste, top with grated Parmesan cheese and fresh basil leaves. Allow it cool for a minute before slicing and serving hot!

## Grilled vegetable quinoa salad

**Ingredients:**

**For Grilled Vegetables:**

- 1 zucchini, sliced lengthwise.

- 1 yellow squash, sliced lengthwise.

- 1 red bell pepper, quartered and deseeded.

- 1 red onion, sliced into thick rings

- 1 cup cherry tomatoes.

- 2 tablespoons of olive oil.

- Salt and pepper to taste.

**For Quinoa:**

- 1 cup quinoa, rinsed.

- 2 cups water or vegetable broth.

- Salt to taste.

**For Salad Dressing:**

- 1/4 cup olive oil.

- 2 tablespoons balsamic vinegar.

- 1 tablespoon honey or maple syrup.

- 1 clove garlic, minced.

- 1 teaspoon Dijon mustard.

- Salt and pepper to taste

**Additional Salad Ingredients:**

- 1/4 cup chopped fresh basil or parsley.

- 1/4 cup crumbled feta cheese or goat cheese (optional).

- 1/4 cup toasted pine nuts or chopped walnuts (optional).

**Instructions:**

**Grilled Vegetables:**

1. Preheat the grill to medium-high heat.

2. Prepare the vegetables: Toss the sliced zucchini, yellow squash, red bell pepper, red onion, and cherry tomatoes with olive oil in a large mixing dish. Season to taste with salt and pepper.

3. Grill veggies: Place the veggies on a hot grill. Grill for 5-7 minutes each side, or until grill marks appear and the meat is tender-crisp. Set aside after removing from the grill.

**Quinoa:**

1. Cook Quinoa: Combine quinoa and water or vegetable broth in a pot. Bring to a boil, then lower to a low heat, cover,

and cook for 15-20 minutes, or until the liquid has been absorbed and the quinoa has been cooked. Allow to cool slightly before fluffing with a fork.

**Salad Dressing:**

1. Make the dressing: In a small mixing bowl, add olive oil, balsamic vinegar, honey or maple syrup, chopped garlic, Dijon mustard, salt, and pepper.

**Assembly:**

1. Combine the ingredients: Combine the cooked quinoa and grilled veggies in a large mixing basin. Drizzle the prepared salad dressing over the mixture and gently toss to evenly cover everything.

2. Add Additional Ingredients: Toss the salad with chopped fresh basil or parsley. To add texture and taste, top with

crumbled feta or goat cheese and toasted pine nuts or chopped walnuts.

3. Chill and Serve: Refrigerate the salad for at least 30 minutes to enable the flavors to mingle. Chill or serve the Grilled Vegetable Quinoa Salad at room temperature.

## Stuffed bell peppers

**Ingredients:**

- 4 large bell peppers (any color).
- 1 cup cooked rice (white or brown).
- 1 pound ground beef or turkey (or substitute with cooked lentils for a vegetarian option).
- 1 small onion, diced.
- 2 cloves garlic, minced.
- 1 can (14 oz) diced tomatoes, drained.
- 1 cup shredded cheese (cheddar, mozzarella, or your choice).

- 1 teaspoon dried oregano.

- 1 teaspoon dried basil.

- Salt and pepper to taste.

- Olive oil for cooking.

**Instructions:**

1. Preheat the oven to 375 degrees F (190 degrees C).

2. Bell Pepper Preparation: Remove the tops of the bell peppers and remove the seeds and membranes. If the peppers don't stand up straight, cut a little bit off the bottom to provide a level surface. Set aside the peppers after rinsing them.

3. Prepare the Filling: Heat a little amount of olive oil in a pan over medium heat. Mix in the diced onions and garlic. Cook for 2-3 minutes, or until aromatic and transparent.

4. Add Ground Meat: To the skillet, add the ground beef or turkey. Cook, breaking it

up with a spoon as it cooks, until it's browned and cooked through.

5. Combine the ingredients: To the pan with the meat, add the cooked rice, drained diced tomatoes, dried oregano, dry basil, salt, and pepper. Stir everything together and simmer for another 3-4 minutes, or until everything is thoroughly blended.

6. Fill the bell peppers with the meat and rice mixture, pushing it very firmly. Place the filled peppers in a baking dish, upright.

7. Bake: Place the baking dish in a preheated oven and cover with foil. 25-30 minutes in the oven.

8. Add Cheese: Remove the foil and top each filled pepper with grated cheese. Return the baking dish, uncovered, to the oven for another 5-7 minutes, or until the cheese is melted and bubbling.

9. Serve: Remove the filled peppers from the oven once done. Allow for a few minutes of cooling before serving. As a filling supper, serve these delectable Stuffed Bell Peppers.

## Lemon garlic shrimp pasta

**Ingredients:**

- 8 ounces of pasta (linguine or spaghetti works well).
- 1 pound of large shrimp, peeled and deveined.
- 4 cloves of garlic, minced.
- Zest of 1 lemon.
- Juice of 1 lemon.
- 2 tablespoons of olive oil.
- 2 tablespoons of butter.
- Salt and pepper to taste.
- Crushed red pepper flakes (optional).
- Chopped fresh parsley for garnish.

* Grated Parmesan cheese (optional).

**Instructions:**

1. Cook the pasta: Boil a big pot of salted water. Cook the pasta until al dente according to package specifications. Reserve 1/2 cup of the cooking water after draining the pasta.

2. Prepare the shrimp by patting them dry with paper towels and seasoning them with salt and pepper.

3. Cook the shrimp: In a large pan over medium-high heat, heat 1 tablespoon olive oil. Cook for 2-3 minutes on each side, or until the shrimp become pink and opaque. Take the shrimp out of the pan and put aside.

4. To make the sauce, heat the remaining olive oil and butter in the same pan.

Cook for about a minute, or until the garlic is aromatic, being careful not to burn it. Stir in the lemon zest and red pepper flakes (if using) for 30 seconds more.

5. Combine everything and turn the heat down low. Add the cooked pasta and lemon juice to the skillet. Toss everything together to properly cover the pasta in the garlic lemon sauce. If the pasta seems dry, gently add part of the conserved pasta water until you achieve the required consistency.

6. Toss in the shrimp: Gently toss in the cooked shrimp to the pasta and sauce, cooking for another minute or two.

7. Remove the skillet from the heat and serve immediately. If necessary, adjust the seasoning with extra salt, pepper, or red pepper flakes. If preferred, garnish

with chopped parsley and grated Parmesan cheese.

8. Serve the Lemon Garlic Shrimp Pasta!

## Chicken pita pockets

**Ingredients:**

- 2 boneless, skinless chicken breasts.

- 1 teaspoon paprika.

- 1 teaspoon garlic powder.

- Salt and pepper to taste.

- 2 tablespoons of olive oil.

- 4 pita bread rounds.

- Toppings (lettuce, tomato, cucumber, red onion, tzatziki sauce, hummus - as desired).

**Instructions:**

1. Prepare the chicken: Thinly slice the chicken breasts. Mix the chicken strips with the paprika, garlic powder, salt, and

pepper in a mixing dish until equally covered.

2. Cook the chicken: In a pan over medium-high heat, heat the olive oil. Cook for 6-8 minutes, or until the seasoned chicken strips are thoroughly cooked through and nicely browned. Stir every now and again to maintain uniform cooking. Remove from the heat once finished.

3. Warm the pita bread: To warm the pita rounds, place them in a toaster, oven, or microwave. This procedure softens them so they may be stuffed.

4. Assemble the pita pockets: Cut pockets into the hot pita bread. Fill the pockets with cooked chicken strips and your favorite toppings like lettuce, tomato, cucumber, red onion, tzatziki sauce, or hummus.

5. To serve, place the filled pita pockets on a dish and serve right away.

## Greek lentil soup

**Ingredients:**

- 1 cup dried green or brown lentils
- 1 onion, finely chopped
- 2 carrots, diced
- 2 celery stalks, diced
- 2 cloves garlic, minced
- 1 can (14 oz) diced tomatoes
- 4 cups vegetable or chicken broth
- 2 tablespoons olive oil
- 1 teaspoon dried oregano
- 1 teaspoon dried thyme
- Salt and pepper to taste
- Optional: Red wine vinegar or lemon juice for serving, crumbled feta cheese, chopped fresh parsley for garnish

**Instructions:**

1. Rinse the lentils: Rinse the lentils in a fine-mesh strainer under cold water and put aside.

2. Saute aromatics: Heat the olive oil in a big saucepan or Dutch oven over medium heat. Mix in the onion, carrots, and celery. 5 minutes, or until the vegetables are softened. Cook for 1 minute more, or until the garlic is fragrant.

3. Add lentils and seasonings: Combine the lentils, diced tomatoes (with liquids), dried oregano, dry thyme, salt, and pepper in a mixing bowl. Pour in the chicken or veggie broth. Bring the ingredients to a boil.

4. Simmer: Once the soup begins to boil, decrease the heat to low and let it simmer, partly covered, for 25-30

minutes, or until the lentils are cooked. Stir every now and again.

5.  Season to taste and serve: Taste the soup and season with extra salt and pepper if necessary. If preferred, add a dash of red wine vinegar or lemon juice for a tangy taste.

6.  Ladle the Greek Lentil Soup into dishes to serve. To enhance flavor and freshness, top each dish with crumbled feta cheese and chopped fresh parsley.

## Grilled veggie sandwich

**Ingredients:**

- 1 zucchini, sliced lengthwise.
- 1 yellow squash, sliced lengthwise.
- 1 red bell pepper, sliced into strips.
- 1 red onion, sliced into rounds.
- 4 slices of bread (sourdough, whole wheat, or your choice).

- 4 tablespoons of olive oil.

- Salt and pepper to taste.

- 1/2 cup of hummus or your preferred spread.

- Handful of fresh spinach or lettuce leaves.

- Optional: Sliced tomatoes, avocado, cheese (like provolone or mozzarella).

## Instructions:

1. Heat the grill or grill pan on medium-high.

2. Toss the zucchini, yellow squash, red bell pepper, and red onion with 2 tablespoons of olive oil in a mixing dish. Season to taste with salt and pepper.

3. Grill the vegetables: Place the vegetables on a hot grill. Grill for 3-4 minutes each side, or until soft and grill marks appear. Set aside after removing from the heat.

4. To toast the bread, brush it with the remaining olive oil. Grill them for approximately a minute on each side, or until gently toasted. Take off the grill.

5. Assemble the sandwich: Spread hummus or your favorite spread on one side of each toasted bread piece. On two pieces of bread, layer the grilled veggies on top of the spread. If preferred, top with fresh spinach or lettuce leaves and any other toppings like sliced tomatoes, avocado, or cheese.

6. Finish the sandwiches: To make sandwiches, top each constructed piece of bread with another slice.

7. Grill the sandwiches: Return the constructed sandwiches to the grill for 2-3 minutes each side, pushing lightly with a spatula, until cooked through and grill marks appear.

8. To serve, remove the grilled vegetable
   sandwiches from the grill and cut them
   in half if preferred.

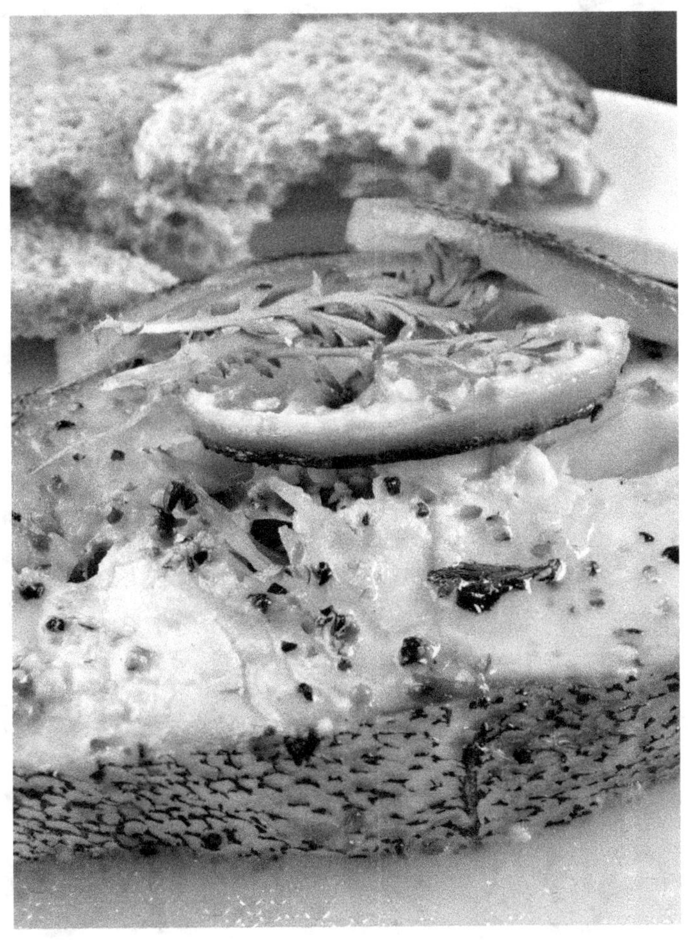

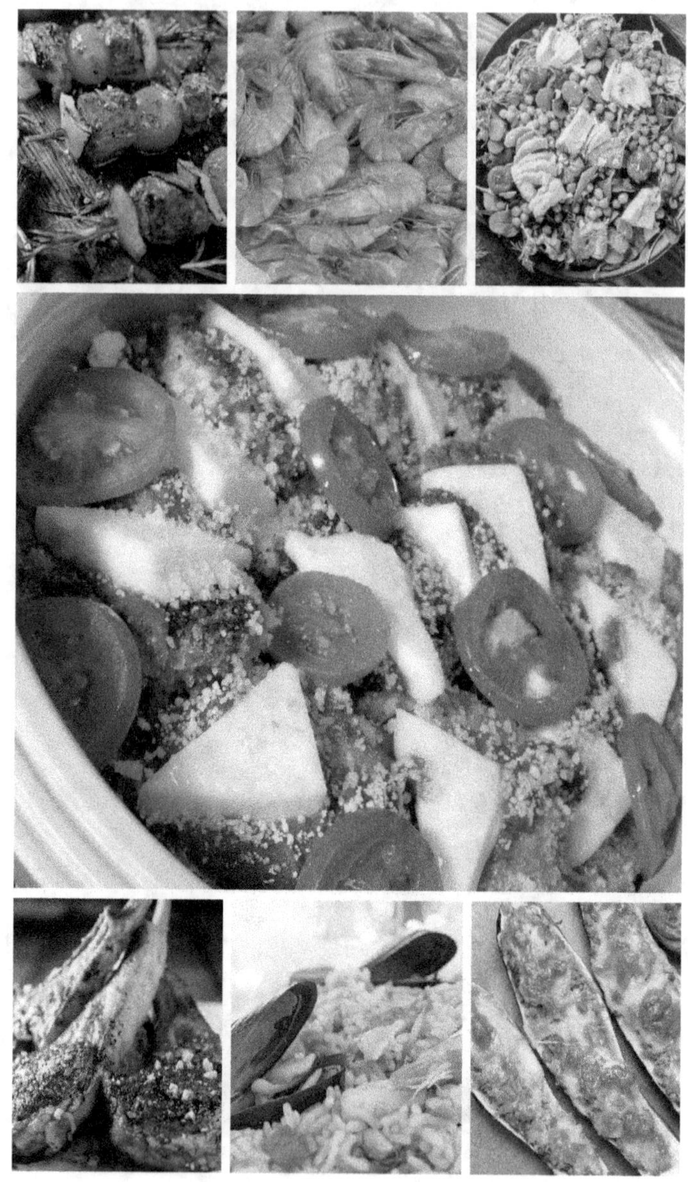

# CHAPTER 4: NOURISHING DINNERS.

## Baked Cod

**Ingredients:**

- 4 cod filets (about 6 ounces each).
- 2 tablespoons of olive oil.
- 2 cloves garlic, minced.
- 1 lemon (zest and juice).
- 1 teaspoon paprika.
- 1 teaspoon dried parsley (or 2 tablespoons chopped fresh parsley).
- Salt and pepper to taste.
- Optional: Sliced lemon for garnish, chopped fresh parsley for garnish.

**Instructions:**

1. Preheat the oven to 400 degrees F (200 degrees C). Line a baking dish with

parchment paper or gently grease it with olive oil.

2. Using paper towels, pat the cod filets dry and set them in the prepared baking dish.

3. Combine the olive oil, minced garlic, lemon zest, lemon juice, paprika, dried parsley (if using fresh parsley, leave it aside for later), salt, and pepper in a small bowl.

4. Drizzle the olive oil mixture evenly over the cod filets, ensuring that they are fully coated on both sides.

5. Optional: Place a slice or two of lemon on top of each filet and sprinkle with more chopped fresh parsley, if preferred.

6. Bake the fish: Preheat the oven to 350°F and bake the baking dish for 12-15 minutes, or until the cod is opaque and flakes readily with a fork.

7. Remove the roasted fish from the oven with care. If preferred, garnish the filets

with more lemon slices or chopped parsley.

## Vegetable paella

**Ingredients:**

- 1 1/2 cups Arborio rice (or short-grain rice).
- 3 cups vegetable broth or vegetable stock.
- 2 tablespoons of olive oil.
- 1 onion, finely chopped.
- 3 cloves garlic, minced.
- 1 red bell pepper, sliced.
- 1 yellow bell pepper, sliced.
- 1 cup cherry tomatoes, halved.
- 1 cup green beans, trimmed and halved.
- 1 teaspoon smoked paprika.
- 1 teaspoon turmeric (for color).
- Pinch of saffron threads (optional).
- Salt and pepper to taste.

- Lemon wedges for serving.
- Chopped fresh parsley for garnish (optional).

**Instructions:**

1. Heat the vegetable broth: In a saucepan over medium heat, cook the vegetable broth. Reduce the heat after it's heated to keep it warm.

2. Prepare the vegetables: Heat the olive oil in a wide, shallow pan or paella pan over medium heat. Sauté the chopped onion and garlic for a few minutes, or until softened.

3. Stir in the vegetables: Add the sliced bell peppers, cherry tomatoes, and green beans. Cook for 5 minutes, or until the veggies soften.

4. Season with smoked paprika, turmeric, and saffron threads (if using) and serve over rice. Stir in the Arborio rice,

making sure it is well coated with the spices and veggies.

5. Pour the soup over the rice and veggies: Carefully pour the heated vegetable broth over the rice and vegetables. Season to taste with salt and pepper. Gently whisk the mixture to properly distribute the ingredients.

6. Simmer and cook: Bring the mixture to a mild boil, then turn it down to a low heat. Allow it to simmer, uncovered, for 20-25 minutes. During this time, avoid stirring the paella to enable the rice to develop a crust on the bottom (known as "socarrat"). Check on a regular basis to check that the liquid has been absorbed and the rice has been cooked.

7. Remove from the fire after the liquid has been absorbed and the rice is tender. Allow the paella to rest for 5-10 minutes,

covered with a clean kitchen cloth or aluminum foil.

8.  Serve: If preferred, garnish the Vegetable Paella with chopped fresh parsley. Serve with lemon wedges for squeezing over the paella before eating.

## Stuffed Zucchini Boats

**Ingredients:**

- 4 medium zucchinis.
- 1 tablespoon of olive oil.
- 1 onion, finely chopped.
- 2 cloves garlic, minced.
- 1 red bell pepper, diced.
- 1 yellow bell pepper, diced.
- 1 cup chopped tomatoes (fresh or canned).
- 1 cup cooked quinoa or rice.
- 1 teaspoon dried oregano.
- 1 teaspoon dried basil.

- Salt and pepper to taste.

- 1/2 cup shredded mozzarella cheese (optional).

- Chopped fresh parsley for garnish (optional).

**Instructions:**

1. Preheat the oven to 375 degrees F (190 degrees C). Grease a baking dish that will contain the zucchini halves.

2. Prepare the zucchinis by cutting them in half lengthwise. Scoop out the seeds and flesh from the middle with a spoon, forming boat-like halves. Around the borders, leave approximately 1/4 inch of flesh. Set aside the zucchini boats that have been hollowed out.

3. To make the filling, chop the zucchini flesh that was removed previously. Warm the olive oil in a pan over medium heat. Mix in the onion, garlic, and diced bell

peppers. Cook for 5 minutes, or until the veggies soften.

4.  Add tomatoes and cooked quinoa/rice: To the pan, add the chopped tomatoes and zucchini flesh. Incorporate the cooked quinoa or rice. Season with oregano, basil, salt, and pepper to taste. Cook for 3-4 minutes more, or until everything is completely mixed and cooked through.

5.  Stuff the zucchini boats: Place the zucchini boats that have been hollowed out in the prepared baking dish. Fill each boat halfway with the vegetable and quinoa/rice mixture, gently pushing it down.

6.  Optional cheese topping: If using, top the packed zucchini boats with shredded mozzarella.

7.  Bake: Place the baking dish in a preheated oven and bake for 20-25

minutes, or until the zucchinis are soft and easily punctured with a fork.

8. To serve, remove the cooked filled zucchini boats from the oven. Garnish with fresh parsley before serving if desired.

## Grilled lamb chops.

**Ingredients:**

- 8 lamb loin chops.
- 2 tablespoons of olive oil.
- 4 cloves garlic, minced.
- 1 tablespoon fresh rosemary, chopped (or 1 teaspoon dried rosemary).
- 1 teaspoon dried thyme.
- Salt and black pepper to taste.
- Optional: Lemon wedges for serving.

**Instructions:**

1. Heat the grill on medium-high.

2.  To make the marinade, combine the olive oil, minced garlic, chopped rosemary, dried thyme, salt, and black pepper in a small bowl.

3.  Coat the lamb chops: Using paper towels, pat the lamb chops dry. Brush the marinade liberally over both sides of the lamb chops.

4.  Rest: Let the lamb chops marinade at room temperature for 20-30 minutes. This allows them to fully absorb the tastes.

5.  Grill the lamb chops: Preheat the grill to medium-high heat. Grill for 3-4 minutes each side for medium-rare doneness, modifying the duration according to your preference.

6.  Rest the lamb chops: When the lamb chops are done, take them from the grill and set them aside for a few minutes

before serving. This distributes the liquids and keeps them wet.

7. To serve, place the cooked lamb chops on a plate. Serve with lemon wedges on the side for a zesty twist.

## Chickpea Salad

**Ingredients:**

- 2 cans (15 ounces each) chickpeas (garbanzo beans), drained and rinsed.
- 1 cucumber, diced.
- 1 bell pepper (any color), diced.
- 1/2 red onion, finely chopped.
- 1 cup cherry tomatoes, halved.
- 1/4 cup chopped fresh parsley.
- 1/4 cup chopped fresh cilantro (optional).
- 1/4 cup olive oil.
- 2 tablespoons red wine vinegar or lemon juice.
- 1 teaspoon dried oregano.

- Salt and pepper to taste.

**Instructions:**

1. Prepare the chickpeas: Drain and thoroughly rinse the canned chickpeas under cold water. Place them in a large mixing basin after petting them dry with a paper towel.

2. Add the vegetables: To the dish containing the chickpeas, add the diced cucumber, bell pepper, red onion, cherry tomatoes, chopped parsley, and cilantro (if using).

3. To make the dressing, mix together the olive oil, red wine vinegar or lemon juice, dried oregano, salt, and pepper in a small bowl.

4. Toss the salad: Pour the dressing over the chickpea and vegetable mixture and toss to combine. Toss everything together

gently until fully blended and uniformly covered with dressing.

5. Chill it: Cover the bowl with plastic wrap or a lid and place the chickpea salad in the refrigerator for at least 30 minutes to enable the flavors to mingle.

6. Toss the salad one last time once it has chilled. Serve the chilled Chickpea Salad as a pleasant side dish or as a light and filling main meal.

## Shrimp and Vegetable Skewers

**Ingredients:**

- 1 pound large shrimp, peeled and deveined.
- 2 bell peppers (any color), cut into chunks.
- 1 red onion, cut into chunks.
- 1 zucchini, sliced into rounds or chunks.
- 1/4 cup olive oil.

- 2 cloves garlic, minced.
- 1 tablespoon lemon juice.
- 1 teaspoon paprika.
- 1 teaspoon dried oregano.
- Salt and pepper to taste.
- Wooden or metal skewers.

**Instructions:**

1. Soak wooden skewers in water for 20-30 minutes before grilling to prevent them from burning.

2. Heat the grill to medium-high.

3. Make the marinade: Whisk together the olive oil, minced garlic, lemon juice, paprika, dried oregano, salt, and pepper in a mixing bowl.

4. Thread the skewers: Thread the shrimp, bell peppers, red onion, and zucchini onto the skewers in alternate directions, producing a mixture of shrimp and veggies on each skewer.

5. Brush the skewers: Arrange the skewers on a dish or tray. Brush the shrimp and veggies with the prepared marinade, making sure they are evenly covered on all sides.

6. Skewers to grill: Place the skewers on the prepared grill. Grill the shrimp for approximately 2-3 minutes each side, or until they are pink and opaque, and the veggies are slightly charred and soft.

7. Serve: Remove the cooked shrimp and veggie skewers from the grill with care. Serve them hot as a tasty and savory appetizer or main course.

## Eggplant Parmesan

**Ingredients:**

- 2 large eggplants.
- Salt.
- 1 cup breadcrumbs.

- 1 cup grated Parmesan cheese.

- 2 eggs, beaten.

- Olive oil for frying.

- 2 cups marinara sauce.

- 2 cups shredded mozzarella cheese.

- Fresh basil leaves for garnish (optional).

**Instructions:**

1. Preheat the oven to 375 degrees F (190 degrees C).

2. Prepare the eggplant: Peel (optional) and slice the eggplants into 1/2-inch circles. Place the slices on paper towels and season both sides. Allow them to sit for approximately 20 minutes to absorb any extra moisture. Using paper towels, pat them dry.

3. Bread the eggplant: Combine the breadcrumbs and grated Parmesan cheese in a shallow dish. In a separate bowl, beat the eggs. Dip each eggplant

slice into the beaten eggs, then coat with the breadcrumb mixture on both sides.

4. Fry the eggplant: Heat the olive oil in a large pan over medium heat. Fry the breaded eggplant slices in batches for 2-3 minutes each side, or until golden brown on both sides. Place the cooked slices on a plate lined with paper towels to absorb any excess oil.

5. Assemble the Eggplant Parmesan: On the bottom of a baking dish, spread a thin layer of marinara sauce. On top of the sauce, stack fried eggplant pieces. More sauce should be poured over the eggplant pieces, and shredded mozzarella cheese should be sprinkled on top. Repeat until all of the eggplant has been utilized, concluding with a layer of sauce and mozzarella cheese on top.

6. Bake: Cover the baking dish with foil and bake for 25-30 minutes, or until the

cheese is melted and bubbling, in a preheated oven.

7. Garnish and serve: Remove the foil from the baking dish and broil for another 2-3 minutes to gently brown the cheese. If preferred, garnish with fresh basil leaves before serving.

# CHAPTER 5: DELECTABLE DESSERTS.

## Greek Yogurt with Honey and Pistachios.

**Ingredients:**

- 1 cup Greek yogurt.
- 2 tablespoons of honey (adjust to taste).
- 2 tablespoons chopped pistachios (or your favorite nuts).

**Instructions:**

1. Place the Greek yogurt in a serving dish or individual serving bowls.
2. Drizzle the yogurt with honey. You may alter the quantity of honey to your desire for sweetness.
3. Scatter the chopped pistachios (or other nuts) over the yogurt and honey.

4. Optional: Top with a dash of cinnamon or a few fresh berries for extra taste and texture.

5. Serve immediately as a healthy breakfast, snack, or dessert with your easy and delicious Greek Yogurt with Honey and Pistachios.

## Baklava.

**Ingredients:**

- 1 package of phyllo pastry sheets (16 ounces)
- 1 1/2 cups chopped nuts (walnuts, pistachios, or a mix)
- 1 cup unsalted butter, melted
- 1 teaspoon ground cinnamon
- 1 cup granulated sugar
- 1 cup water
- 1/2 cup honey
- 1 teaspoon vanilla extract

**Instructions:**

1. Preheat the oven to 350 degrees Fahrenheit (175 degrees Celsius). Grease a baking dish (often 9x13 inches) with butter.
2. Thaw frozen phyllo pastry according per package directions. To keep it from drying out, cover it with a moist towel.
3. In a mixing dish, combine the chopped nuts and ground cinnamon.
4. Line a baking dish with one piece of phyllo pastry. Brush it with melted butter liberally. Repeat the stacking and buttering procedure until you've used up approximately half of the phyllo sheets.
5. Evenly distribute half of the nut mixture over the stacked phyllo sheets.
6. Layer the remaining phyllo sheets on top of the nut mixture, buttering each sheet as you go.

7. Scatter the leftover nut mixture on top of the phyllo sheets.

8. Cut the baklava into diamond or square shapes using a sharp knife.

9. Bake for 45-50 minutes, or until the baklava is golden brown, in a preheated oven.

10. Make the syrup while the baklava is baking. Combine the granulated sugar, water, honey, and vanilla essence in a saucepan. Bring the mixture to a mild boil, then lower to a low heat and allow it simmer for 10-15 minutes, or until it thickens slightly to a syrupy consistency.

11. Remove the baklava from the oven and quickly pour the hot syrup over the heated baklava, making sure it covers all of the cut lines.

12. Remove the baklava from the baking dish and set aside to cool fully. This

permits the syrup to go deeper into the layers.

13. Lastly, serve and enjoy your handmade Baklava! Any leftovers should be stored in an airtight jar at room temperature.

## Orange and Almond cake.

**Ingredients:**

- 3 large oranges
- 6 eggs
- 1 cup granulated sugar
- 2 cups almond meal (ground almonds)
- 1 teaspoon baking powder
- Powdered sugar for dusting (optional)

**Instructions:**

1. Preheat the oven to 350 degrees Fahrenheit (175 degrees Celsius). Grease and line a 9-inch-diameter round cake pan with parchment paper.

2. Thoroughly wash the oranges. Put them in a pot hole and cover with water. Bring the water to a boil, then decrease the heat and let the oranges simmer for 1-1.5 hours, or until very soft. Drain and set aside to cool.

3. Once the oranges have cooled, cut them into quarters, remove any seeds, and purée them in a blender or food processor (with the skin) until smooth.

4. In a mixing basin, whisk together the eggs and granulated sugar until thoroughly blended.

5. Stir in the almond meal, baking powder, and orange puree to the egg mixture. Mix until everything is well blended.

6. Pour the batter into the cake pan that has been prepared.

7. Bake for 50-60 minutes in a preheated oven, or until a toothpick inserted into the middle of the cake comes out clean.

8. Remove the cake from the oven and cool it in the pan for approximately 10-15 minutes. After that, place it on a wire rack to cool entirely.

9. Optional: Before serving, dust the top of the cooled cake with powdered sugar.

10. Cut and serve your delicious Orange and Almond Cake! The cake is moist and tasty, with a nice citrusy note from the oranges and nutty richness from the almonds.

## Ricotta and Honey Stuffed Figs.

**Ingredients:**

- 8 fresh figs.
- 1/2 cup ricotta cheese.
- 2 tablespoons of honey (plus extra for drizzling).
- 1/4 teaspoon ground cinnamon.

- 2 tablespoons chopped nuts (such as walnuts or pistachios), optional.
- Fresh mint leaves for garnish, optional.

**Instructions:**

1. Preheat the oven to 350 degrees Fahrenheit (175 degrees Celsius).
2. Wash and dry the figs with a paper towel. Remove the stem end of each fig and make a tiny cross-shaped incision halfway down the top of each fig to create an aperture for filling.
3. In a mixing dish, combine the ricotta cheese, honey, and ground cinnamon.
4. Gently open each fig and pour a little quantity of the ricotta mixture into each fig's middle.
5. Optional: For extra texture and taste, sprinkle the chopped nuts over the filled figs.

6. Arrange the filled figs on a parchment-lined baking sheet.

7. Bake for 10-12 minutes, or until the figs are slightly softened and the ricotta mixture is warmed through, in a preheated oven.

8. Remove the filled figs from the oven and set aside for a few minutes to cool.

9. Just before serving, drizzle the packed figs with a little additional honey.

10. For a flash of color and additional freshness, garnish with fresh mint leaves.

## Fruit salad.

**Ingredients:**

- Assorted fresh fruits (such as strawberries, blueberries, grapes, pineapple, melon, oranges, kiwi, etc.), washed and chopped.

- 2 tablespoons honey (optional, for added sweetness).
- Juice of 1 lemon or lime (for a citrusy touch).
- Fresh mint leaves for garnish (optional)

**Instructions:**

1. Prepare the fruits: Thoroughly wash all of the fruits and cut them into bite-sized pieces. You may use any mix of fruits you choose or whatever is in season.
2. Toss the chopped fruits in a large mixing dish.
3. Drizzle the honey over the mixed fruits if desired for extra sweetness. Instead of or in addition to the honey, pour the juice of a lemon or lime over the fruits if you like a tart taste.
4. Gently toss the fruits in the honey or citrus juice to coat evenly.

5. Optional: For an added blast of flavor and freshness, garnish the fruit salad with fresh mint leaves.

6. Refrigerate the fruit salad for 15-30 minutes before serving to enable the flavors to mingle.

7. For a refreshing and nutritious treat, serve your delightful Fruit Salad in individual bowls or as a side dish!


## Lemon semolina cake.

**Ingredients:**
- 1 cup fine semolina
- 1 cup plain yogurt
- 1 cup granulated sugar
- 1/2 cup vegetable oil
- Zest of 2 lemons
- Juice of 1 lemon
- 1 teaspoon baking powder

- 1/2 teaspoon baking soda

- Pinch of salt

- Powdered sugar for dusting (optional)

## Instructions:

1. Preheat the oven to 350 degrees Fahrenheit (175 degrees Celsius). Grease and flour an 8 or 9-inch-diameter round cake pan, or line it with parchment paper.

2. Combine the fine semolina, plain yogurt, granulated sugar, and vegetable oil in a mixing dish. Mix until everything is properly blended.

3. Add the lemon zest and juice to the mixture and stir well.

4. Add the baking powder, baking soda, and salt to taste. Blend until the batter is smooth and everything is combined.

5. Pour the batter into the cake pan that has been prepared.

6. Bake for 30-35 minutes, or until the cake is golden brown and a toothpick inserted into the middle comes out clean, in a preheated oven.

7. Remove the cake from the oven and cool it in the pan for approximately 10-15 minutes.

8. Carefully remove the cake from the oven and place it on a wire rack to cool entirely.

9. Optional: Before serving, dust the top of the cooled cake with powdered sugar for decorating.

10. Slice and serve your wonderful Lemon Semolina Cake! The lemon zest and juice provide a delightful zesty zing to this delicious and delectable cake.

## Date and Nut Bars.

**Ingredients:**

- 1 cup pitted dates.
- 1 cup mixed nuts (such as almonds, walnuts, pecans).
- 1/2 cup rolled oats.
- 2 tablespoons honey or maple syrup.
- Pinch of salt.
- Optional add-ins: 1/2 teaspoon vanilla extract, 1/2 teaspoon cinnamon.

**Instructions:**

1. Preheat the oven to 350 degrees Fahrenheit (175 degrees Celsius). Line a baking dish or pan with parchment paper, allowing enough overhang for subsequent removal.
2. Prepare the dates: Soak the dates in boiling water for 10-15 minutes, then drain well. This softens them and prepares them for mixing.
3. Process the dates, mixed nuts, rolled oats, honey or maple syrup, and a bit of

salt in a food processor until a sticky, gritty mixture forms. If using, add optional vanilla extract or cinnamon and pulse to blend.

4. Press into baking dish: Place the mixture in the prepared baking dish. Press the mixture firmly and evenly into the pan with a spatula or your fingertips.

5. Bake: Bake for 15-20 minutes, or until the edges are slightly brown, in a preheated oven.

6. Cool and cut: Remove the pan from the oven after baking and allow the date and nut mixture to cool fully in the pan. When the block has cooled, take it out of the pan using the parchment paper overhang. Place it on a cutting board and cut it into squares or bars.

7. Serve and store: You can eat your homemade Date and Nut Bars right away

or keep them in an airtight jar at room temperature for up to a week.

## Rice Pudding (Rizogalo)

**Ingredients:**

- 1/2 cup Arborio rice (or any short-grain rice).
- 4 cups of whole milk.
- 1/2 cup sugar.
- 1 cinnamon stick (or 1 teaspoon ground cinnamon).
- 1 teaspoon vanilla extract (optional)
- Pinch of salt.
- Ground cinnamon for garnish (optional).

**Instructions:**

1. Rinse the rice: Rinse the rice in a fine-mesh strainer under cold water and put it aside.

2. Cook the rice: In a large saucepan over medium heat, mix the milk and washed rice. Add the cinnamon stick (ground cinnamon may be added afterward). Bring the mixture to a mild boil, stirring regularly to keep the rice from sticking to the pan's bottom.

3. Simmer: Reduce the heat to low after the milk begins to boil. Allow the rice to simmer, uncovered, for 25-30 minutes, or until the rice is tender and the sauce thickens. If used, remove the cinnamon stick.

4. To sweeten the pudding, combine the sugar, vanilla extract (if using), and a touch of salt in a mixing bowl. Continue to cook for 5-10 minutes, stirring regularly, until the sugar melts and the pudding achieves the desired consistency.

5. Remove from the fire and set aside for a few minutes to cool before serving. If you want it cold, let it cool entirely in the refrigerator before serving.

6. Garnish and serve: If preferred, add powdered cinnamon on top of each dish before serving.

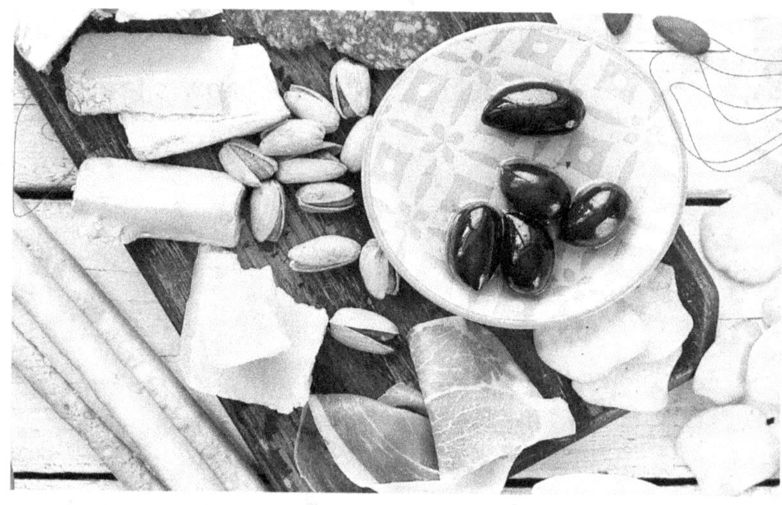

# CHAPTER 6: WELLNESS BEYOND THE PLATE.

Beyond the plate investigates several areas of wellness that contribute to a healthy lifestyle other than eating habits. It dives into important aspects such as physical exercise, mental health, sleep, and stress management.

Physical activity is essential for general well-being. It does not have to be strenuous exercise; simple activities such as walking, yoga, or dancing might help. Movement in your everyday routine improves flexibility, strength, and cardiovascular health.

Mental Health: Wellness entails caring for your mind as well as your body. Stress management techniques, finding moments of relaxation, practicing mindfulness or meditation, and getting help when required all contribute to mental health.

Sleep: Adequate sleep is essential for general health. You must comprehend the necessity of developing healthy sleeping habits, creating a tranquil sleeping environment, and comprehending the relevance of excellent sleep for physical and mental health.

Stress Management: Stress has a variety of effects on health. It is critical for general wellbeing to learn how to handle stress via relaxation methods, time management, establishing boundaries, and engaging in activities that offer pleasure and tranquility.

# CONCLUSION.

## Conversion Charts

Length:

- 1 inch = 2.54 centimeters
- 1 foot = 30.48 centimeters
- 1 meter = 3.28 feet
- 1 mile = 1.61 kilometers

Weight:

- 1 pound = 0.45 kilograms
- 1 kilogram = 2.20 pounds
- 1 ounce = 28.35 grams
- 

Volume:

- 1 gallon = 3.78 liters
- 1 liter = 0.26 gallons
- 1 cup = 236.59 milliliters

Temperature:

- Celsius to Fahrenheit: $F = (C \times 9/5) + 32$
- Fahrenheit to Celsius: $C = (F - 32) \times 5/9$

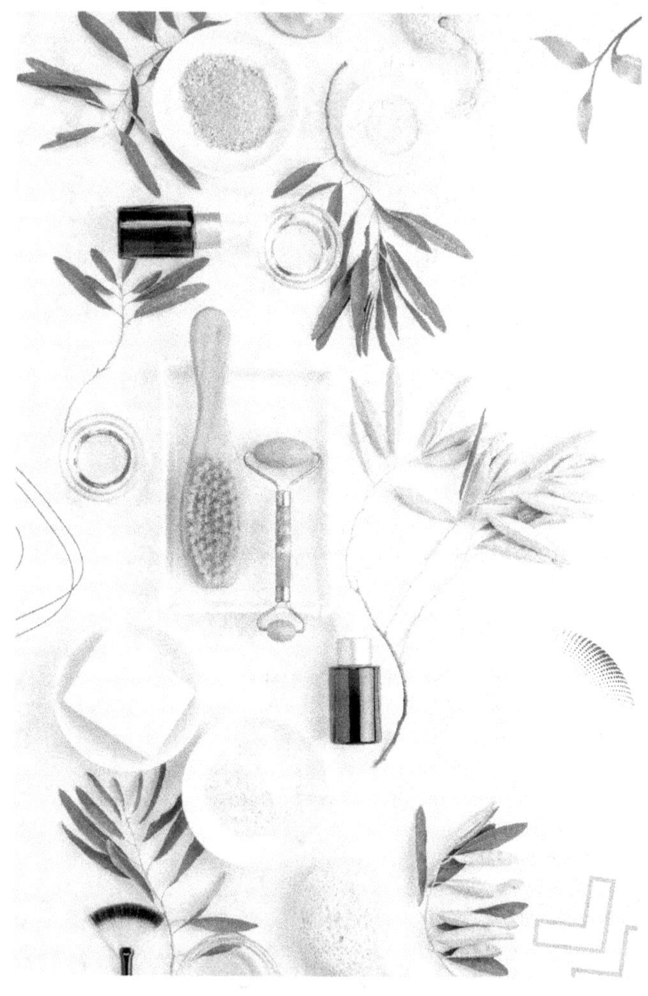

# ADDITIONAL RESOURCES.

Exploring the Mediterranean diet is more than simply a recipe; it's an invitation to a way of life rich in health advantages and gastronomic pleasures. For couples looking to embark on this fascinating trip together, a plethora of websites provide an abundance of recipes, advice, and inspiration to make this culinary excursion a memorable one.

Cookbooks: A treasure trove of Mediterranean-inspired cookbooks caters exclusively to couples looking to start on a culinary health journey. Look for literature on the Mediterranean. These publications often provide simple recipes, portion sizes suitable for two people, and helpful hints for integrating Mediterranean foods into regular meals.

Online Recipe Databases: There are several websites and gourmet blogs that have a large variety of Mediterranean recipes designed for couples. Websites devoted to healthy cooking often organize sections or filters expressly for two-serving recipes. These platforms provide a wide range of recipes, from fast and simple workday meals to romantic date-night dinners, making it easy to experiment with new tastes and cooking methods.

Meal Subscription Services: Several meal subscription services provide fresh ingredients and Mediterranean-inspired dishes to your home. Choose subscription boxes created for two-person servings, which enable couples to experiment with tastes and ingredients while also enjoying the convenience of pre-portioned meals without the effort of grocery shopping.

Cooking lessons and Workshops: Participating in cooking lessons or workshops geared toward Mediterranean food may be a fun and participatory method for couples to learn together. Many culinary schools and community organizations provide lessons on Mediterranean cooking methods and dishes. These courses not only teach culinary skills but also allow couples to connect while creating and enjoying meals together.

Social media platforms and YouTube channels devoted to food and wellness often include influencers or chefs specialized in Mediterranean cuisine. Following these accounts gives couples access to a plethora of recipe ideas, culinary advice, and video demonstrations, making it simple to recreate delectable Mediterranean delicacies in their own kitchen.

Mobile Apps: Explore a plethora of mobile apps specialized to Mediterranean cuisine and meal planning. These applications make it simple for couples to browse recipes, make shopping lists, and plan meals together. Some applications even allow for dietary modification and include interactive elements for monitoring nutritional intake.

Exploring local food markets and ethnic shops may be a pleasant excursion for couples looking for real Mediterranean foods. These markets often provide a diverse selection of fresh vegetables, spices, olives, cheeses, and other ingredients, enabling couples to explore and experiment with authentic Mediterranean tastes in their recipes.

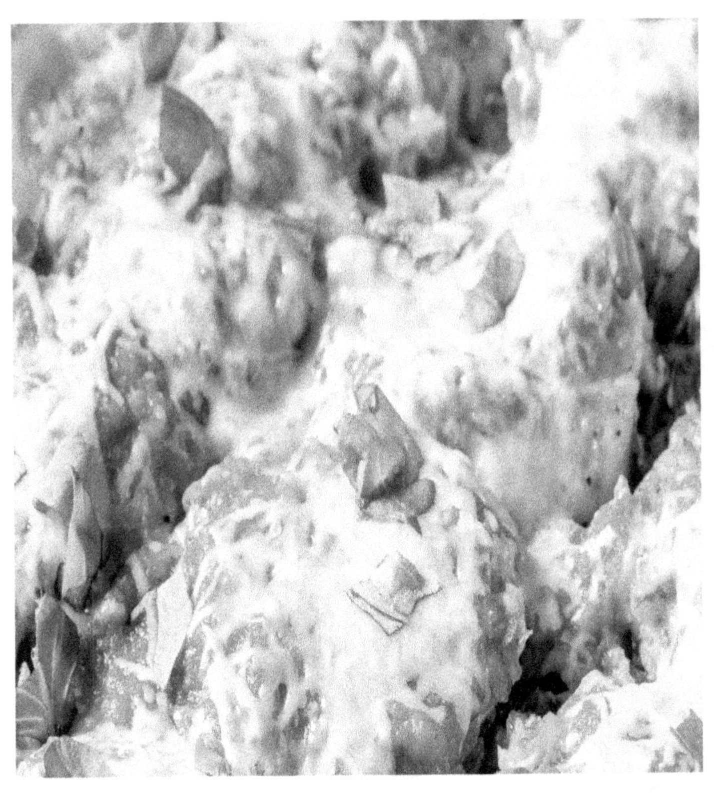